Bodybuilding Workout Diet Plan for Women

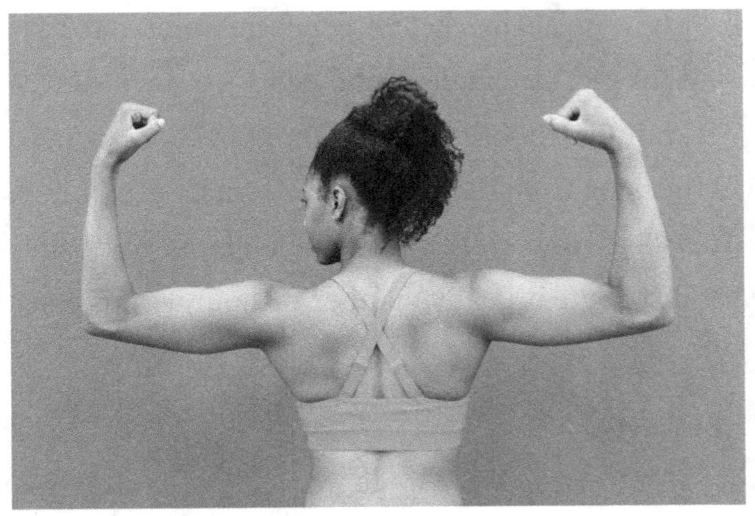

A Comprehensive Meal Plan for Muscle Gain in Women

Patrick Moore

Table of Contents

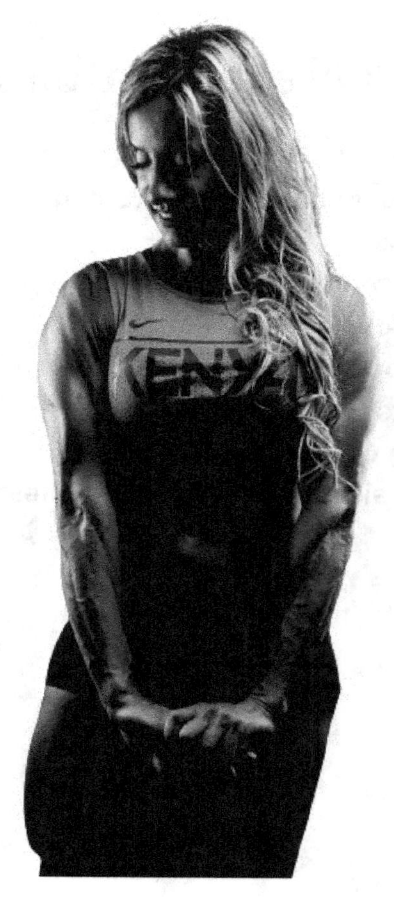

Introduction

Welcome to "Strong and Sculpted: The Ultimate Bodybuilding Workout Diet Plan for Women"! This book is your comprehensive guide to unlocking your full potential and achieving a strong, fit, and beautifully sculpted physique through the power of bodybuilding.

For too long, the realm of bodybuilding has been dominated by men, leaving women feeling excluded or unsure of how to navigate their own fitness journey. But times have changed, and this book is here to empower you with the knowledge, strategies, and practical tips tailored specifically to the unique needs and goals of women in the world of bodybuilding.

Bodybuilding is not about conforming to societal expectations or fitting into a mold. It's about embracing your strength, celebrating your body, and pushing beyond your limits to achieve the extraordinary. Whether you're a complete beginner or an experienced fitness enthusiast, this book will provide you with the roadmap to build lean muscle, increase strength, and transform your physique.

In the pages ahead, we will dive deep into the foundational principles of bodybuilding for women. You'll discover the countless benefits that await you on this transformative journey, dispel common myths and misconceptions, and learn how to overcome the challenges that may arise along the way.

Nutrition is a cornerstone of bodybuilding success, and we will guide you in creating a diet plan that supports your goals. You'll explore the essential macronutrients and micronutrients needed for muscle growth and recovery, learn how to calculate your caloric needs, and master the art of meal planning and prepping.

Designing an effective workout plan is equally crucial, and we will provide you with expert guidance to develop a routine that combines resistance training, cardiovascular exercise, and proper rest and recovery. From beginner to advanced levels, you'll find customizable workout programs designed to optimize your progress and keep you motivated.

As we delve into the world of bodybuilding supplements, we will demystify their role and provide recommendations for safe and effective supplementation tailored specifically for women.

But bodybuilding is not just about the physical aspect; it's a holistic journey that encompasses the mind, body, and soul. We will address common challenges such as plateaus, maintaining motivation, and dealing with body image issues. Moreover, we will explore how to build a sustainable lifestyle and create healthy habits that will ensure long-term success.

Throughout this book, you'll find practical tips, inspiring success stories, and the knowledge to take control of your bodybuilding journey. You have the power to shape your physique, improve your confidence, and redefine what it means to be strong and sculpted as a woman.

Are you ready to embark on this transformative adventure? Let's dive in and unlock the extraordinary potential within you. Your strong and sculpted future starts now!

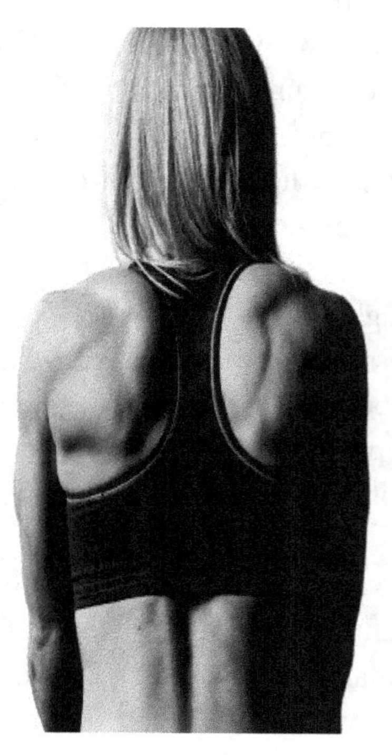

Benefits of Bodybuilding for Women

Bodybuilding is often associated with men, with images of bulging muscles and intense strength dominating the perception. However, bodybuilding holds a multitude of benefits for women as well. Embracing the world of bodybuilding can empower women in numerous ways, positively impacting both their physical and mental well-being. Here are some key benefits of bodybuilding specifically tailored for women:

1. Strength and Muscle Development: Engaging in bodybuilding workouts allows women to develop strength and build lean muscle mass. Contrary to common misconceptions, weightlifting and resistance training do not lead to bulky muscles in women. Instead, bodybuilding exercises help sculpt a well-defined physique, enhancing muscle tone and creating a lean, strong, and feminine appearance.

2. Increased Metabolism: Building muscle through bodybuilding can significantly increase your metabolic rate. As muscles require more energy to maintain than fat, the development of lean muscle mass boosts your resting metabolic rate. This means that even when you are at rest, your body continues to burn more calories, assisting in weight management and supporting a healthy body composition.

3. Improved Bone Health: Women are more susceptible to osteoporosis and bone-related issues as they age. Bodybuilding exercises, especially weight-bearing exercises, help promote bone density and strength. By challenging your bones through resistance training, you stimulate the production of new bone tissue, reducing the risk of fractures and osteoporosis.

4. Enhanced Body Composition: Bodybuilding allows women to reshape their bodies by reducing body fat and increasing muscle mass. Through a combination of proper nutrition and targeted workouts, bodybuilding promotes a favourable body composition, helping you achieve a leaner and more defined physique. This can boost self-confidence, body image, and overall well-being.

5. Increased Strength and Functional Fitness: Bodybuilding workouts improve not only muscular strength but also functional fitness. Functional fitness focuses on enhancing your ability to perform everyday activities with ease and efficiency. Whether it's lifting heavy objects, carrying groceries, or participating in recreational sports, bodybuilding exercises enhance your overall strength and physical capabilities, making daily life tasks easier.

6. Improved Hormonal Balance: Bodybuilding can positively impact hormonal balance in women. Engaging in regular exercise, especially strength training, can help regulate hormone levels, including estrogen and progesterone. This can have beneficial effects on menstrual health, reduce symptoms of premenstrual syndrome (PMS), and contribute to overall hormonal well-being.

7. Mental and Emotional Empowerment: Bodybuilding is not just about physical transformations; it also provides a platform for mental and emotional growth. The discipline, dedication, and perseverance required in bodybuilding can foster mental resilience and fortitude. Achieving fitness goals, overcoming challenges, and witnessing personal progress can boost self-confidence, self-esteem, and a sense of empowerment.

8. Stress Relief and Mental Well-being: Exercise, including bodybuilding, is a proven stress-reliever and mood enhancer. Engaging in physical activity releases endorphins, the body's natural mood-elevating chemicals, promoting feelings of well-being and reducing stress levels. Bodybuilding can serve as a productive outlet for stress, allowing you to channel your energy into something positive while benefiting both your body and mind.

9. Long-Term Health Benefits: Regular bodybuilding exercises contribute to long-term health and disease prevention. It helps reduce the risk of chronic conditions such as cardiovascular diseases, type 2 diabetes, and certain types of cancer. By maintaining a strong, healthy body through bodybuilding, women can enjoy a higher quality of life and improved overall health in the years to come.

Setting Goals

Setting clear and achievable goals is a fundamental step in any bodybuilding journey. Goals provide direction, motivation, and a roadmap to track progress. Whether you're a beginner or an experienced athlete, defining your objectives is crucial to staying focused and committed. Here are some key points to consider when setting goals for your bodybuilding endeavors:

1. Specificity: Your goals should be specific and well-defined. Rather than a vague goal like "getting in shape," consider more precise targets such as reducing body fat percentage, increasing muscle mass in specific areas, or achieving a certain strength milestone. Specific goals provide clarity and allow you to create a focused plan of action.

2. Realistic and Attainable: While it's important to challenge yourself, it's equally important to set goals that are realistic and attainable. Be honest with yourself about your current fitness level, available time, and resources. Setting unrealistic goals can lead to frustration and demotivation. Start with smaller, achievable goals and gradually progress from there.

3. Time-Bound: Establishing a timeline for your goals adds a sense of urgency and accountability. Consider setting both short-term and long-term goals. Short-term goals could be weekly or monthly targets, while long-term goals may span several months or even years. Breaking down your goals into smaller, manageable increments helps track progress and maintain motivation.

4. Measurable: It's essential to have measurable goals to track your progress objectively. Measurable goals allow you to monitor your performance and determine if you're moving in the right direction. This could involve tracking parameters like body weight, body fat percentage, strength gains, or specific exercise performance. Use tools such as body measurements, progress photos, or fitness apps to help measure and visualise your progress.

5. Personalization: Your goals should be tailored to your individual needs, preferences, and aspirations. Avoid comparing yourself to others or setting goals solely based on societal expectations. Understand your unique starting point, body type, and desired outcomes. Focus on improving your own performance and becoming the best version of yourself.

6. Long-Term Vision: While setting short-term goals is essential for immediate progress, it's equally important to have a long-term vision. Envision the ultimate outcome you desire and use it as a guiding light. Having a long-term vision helps maintain perspective during challenging times and allows you to make decisions aligned with your larger goals.

7. Flexibility and Adaptability: Recognize that goals may need to be adjusted along the way. As you progress, your circumstances and priorities may change. Be open to adapting your goals as needed while staying true to your overall vision. Embrace the journey and be willing to modify your approach based on new insights or unexpected obstacles.

8. Accountability and Support: Share your goals with trusted friends, family members, or a coach who can provide support and hold you accountable. Communicating your goals makes them more tangible and helps create a support system. Regular check-ins, progress updates, or joining a fitness community can provide the encouragement and guidance needed to stay on track.

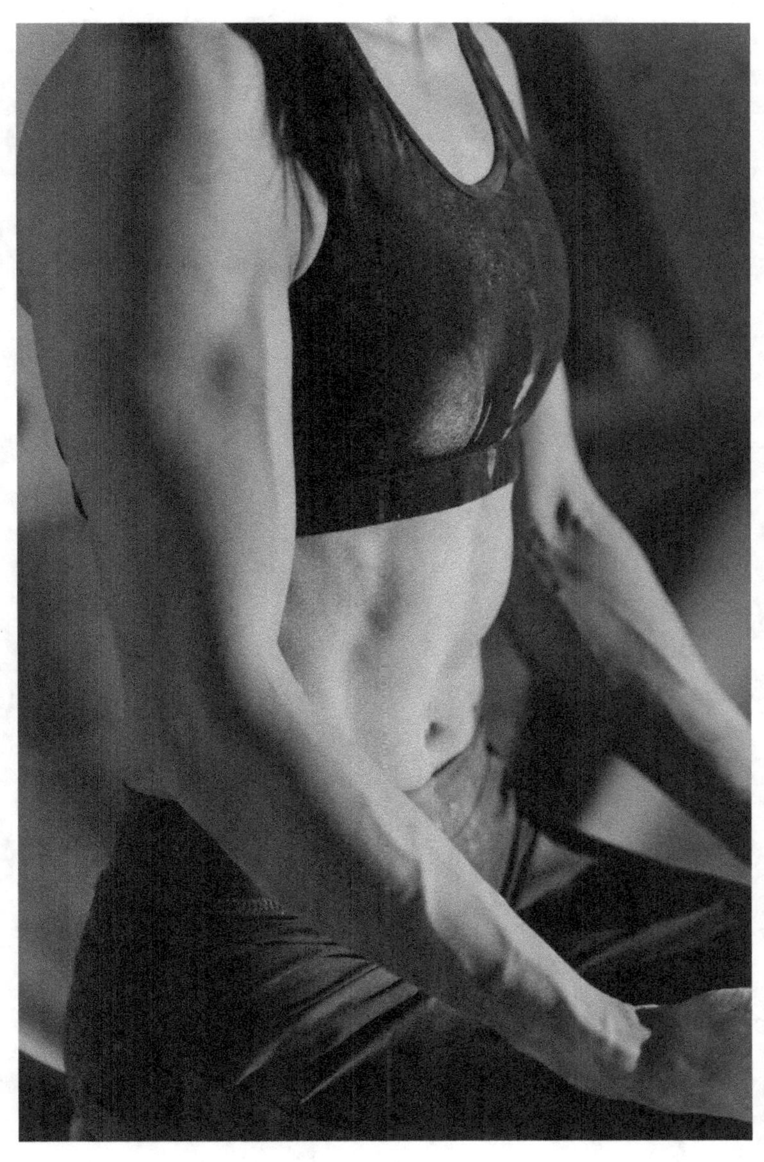

Nutrition Essentials

Proper nutrition is a cornerstone of bodybuilding success. It provides the essential building blocks for muscle growth, supports recovery, and optimizes overall health. Understanding nutrition fundamentals and implementing a well-balanced diet plan is crucial for achieving your bodybuilding goals. Here are some key nutrition essentials to consider:

1. Macronutrients: Macronutrients are the primary components of your diet and include proteins, carbohydrates, and fats.

   - *Proteins:* Protein is vital for muscle repair and growth. Aim to include high-quality protein sources such as lean meats, poultry, fish, eggs, dairy, legumes, and plant-based proteins like tofu or tempeh. Distribute protein intake evenly throughout the day to support muscle synthesis.

   - *Carbohydrates:* Carbohydrates provide the energy needed for intense workouts and replenish glycogen stores. Focus on complex carbohydrates like whole grains, fruits, vegetables, and legumes. Prioritize nutrient-dense options over processed or refined carbohydrates.

- *Fats:* Healthy fats are essential for hormone production, nutrient absorption, and overall health. Include sources of unsaturated fats like avocados, nuts, seeds, olive oil, and fatty fish. Moderate your intake of saturated and trans fats found in processed foods and fried items.

2. Micronutrients: Micronutrients, including vitamins and minerals, play vital roles in various bodily functions. Consume a variety of fruits, vegetables, whole grains, and nuts to ensure an adequate intake of micronutrients. Consider a balanced multivitamin or consult with a registered dietitian if you have specific nutrient deficiencies.

3. Caloric Balance: To support your bodybuilding goals, it's crucial to maintain a caloric balance that aligns with your objectives.

- *Caloric Surplus:* If your goal is to build muscle mass, you may need to consume a slight caloric surplus. This means consuming more calories than you burn, typically achieved through a combination of increased portion sizes and additional snacks or meals.

- Caloric Deficit: **If your goal is to reduce body fat, creating a caloric deficit is necessary. This involves consuming fewer calories than you burn. Gradually reduce calorie intake through portion control, mindful eating, and choosing nutrient-dense foods.**

- Tracking and Adjusting: **Tracking your food intake using apps or journals can help monitor your caloric balance. Regularly assess your progress and adjust your calorie intake based on your goals and individual needs.**

4. Meal Planning and Timing: Meal planning and timing can optimise nutrient availability and support your workouts.

- Pre-Workout Nutrition: Consume a balanced meal or snack containing carbohydrates and protein 1-3 hours before your workout to provide sustained energy and support muscle performance.

- Post-Workout Nutrition: After exercise, prioritise a meal or snack containing protein and carbohydrates to aid in muscle recovery and glycogen replenishment.

- Meal Frequency: The frequency of meals and snacks can vary based on personal preference and schedule. Aim for a consistent pattern of eating, including a

combination of whole food meals and balanced snacks to maintain energy levels and support muscle growth.

5. Hydration: Proper hydration is essential for overall health and optimal performance.

- *Water:* Aim to drink plenty of water throughout the day, especially during workouts. Staying hydrated supports digestion, nutrient absorption, muscle function, and helps regulate body temperature.

- *Electrolytes:* During intense workouts or in hot climates, electrolytes may need to be replenished. Consider incorporating electrolyte-rich beverages or supplements to maintain balance.

6. Individualization and Flexibility: Nutrition needs vary among individuals. Listen to your body and adjust your diet accordingly. Experiment with different approaches and foods to find what works best for you. Consulting with a registered dietitian can provide personalised guidance and ensure your nutritional needs are met.

Designing Your Workout Plan

Designing an effective workout plan is essential for achieving your bodybuilding goals. A well-structured and balanced training program will help you build muscle, increase strength, improve endurance, and shape your physique. Here are key factors to consider when designing your workout plan:

1. Define Your Goals: Start by clarifying your specific goals. Do you want to build overall muscle mass, focus on specific muscle groups, increase strength, or improve athletic performance? Defining your goals will guide your exercise selection, set-rep scheme, and overall training approach.

2. Resistance Training: Incorporate resistance training as the foundation of your workout plan. This involves using weights, resistance bands, or bodyweight exercises to challenge your muscles. Focus on compound exercises that target multiple muscle groups, such as squats, deadlifts, bench presses, and pull-ups. Include both free weights and machines to provide variety and target different muscle fibers.

3. Split or Full-Body: Determine whether you prefer a split routine or a full-body workout approach. Split routines involve dividing your training sessions into specific muscle groups or body parts, training them on separate days. Full-body workouts engage the entire body in each session. Choose the approach that aligns with your goals, schedule, and recovery capacity.

4. Frequency and Rest Days: Consider how many days per week you can commit to training. Aim for a minimum of 3-4 sessions per week to allow adequate stimulus for muscle growth and recovery. Include rest days between training sessions to promote muscle repair and prevent overtraining. Listen to your body and adjust the frequency and rest days as needed.

5. Volume and Intensity: Volume refers to the total workload performed during a training session, including sets, reps, and weights. Intensity refers to the level of effort and resistance used. Find the right balance of volume and intensity that challenges your muscles without risking injury or excessive fatigue. Gradually increase the volume and intensity over time to stimulate ongoing progress.

6. Progressive Overload: Incorporate the principle of progressive overload to continually challenge your muscles and stimulate growth. This involves gradually increasing the demands on your muscles by adding weight, increasing reps, or reducing rest time. Keep a training log to track your progress and ensure you're consistently pushing your limits.

7. Cardiovascular Exercise: While resistance training is the primary focus of bodybuilding, cardiovascular exercise contributes to overall fitness and health. Include cardiovascular workouts, such as jogging, cycling, or swimming, to improve cardiovascular endurance and aid in fat loss. The frequency and duration of cardiovascular exercise depend on your goals and preferences.

8. Flexibility and Mobility: Don't overlook the importance of flexibility and mobility. Incorporate dynamic warm-ups, stretching, and mobility exercises to improve joint range of motion, prevent injuries, and enhance overall movement quality. Consider including dedicated flexibility or yoga sessions to support recovery and maintain flexibility.

9. Periodization: Implement periodization to structure your training plan into different phases or cycles. Periodization involves alternating between periods of higher intensity and lower intensity, varying the training variables to prevent plateau and optimize progress. This can include changing rep ranges, adjusting weights, or modifying exercises.

10. Seek Professional Guidance: If you're new to bodybuilding or unsure about designing your own workout plan, consider seeking guidance from a certified personal trainer or strength and conditioning specialist. They can provide expert advice, assess your specific needs, and design a customised program tailored to your goals, abilities, and any existing limitations.

Workout Programs for Women

Women have unique fitness goals and considerations, and workout programs designed specifically for them can help maximise results and promote overall well-being. Whether your aim is to build strength, increase endurance, improve flexibility, or enhance body composition, here are some key elements to consider when designing a workout program for women:

1. Resistance Training: Incorporate resistance training to build strength, increase lean muscle mass, and improve overall body composition. Focus on compound exercises that target multiple muscle groups, such as squats, lunges, deadlifts, push-ups, rows, and overhead presses. Use a variety of equipment, including free weights, resistance bands, and machines, to provide versatility and challenge different muscle fibers.

2. Cardiovascular Exercise: Include cardiovascular workouts to improve cardiovascular health, boost endurance, and support fat loss. Engage in activities such as jogging, cycling, swimming, or high-intensity interval training (HIIT). Find activities that you enjoy to make cardio sessions more enjoyable and sustainable.

3. Core and Stability Training: Strengthening the core muscles is essential for overall stability, balance, and injury prevention. Incorporate exercises like planks, Russian twists, bird dogs, and stability ball exercises to target the core muscles effectively. Developing core strength can also enhance posture and contribute to a toned and sculpted midsection.

4. Flexibility and Mobility: Prioritise flexibility and mobility exercises to maintain joint range of motion, prevent injuries, and improve overall movement quality. Incorporate dynamic warm-ups, stretching routines, and exercises that promote mobility, such as yoga or Pilates. Focus on stretching major muscle groups and areas prone to tightness, such as hips, hamstrings, shoulders, and chest.

5. High-Intensity Interval Training (HIIT): HIIT workouts involve alternating between high-intensity bursts of exercise and short recovery periods. This time-efficient approach can help burn calories, boost metabolism, and improve cardiovascular fitness. Choose exercises that work multiple muscle groups, such as squat jumps, burpees, mountain climbers, and kettlebell swings, to maximise the effectiveness of HIIT workouts.

6. Mind-Body Activities: Incorporate mind-body activities like yoga, tai chi, or meditation to promote relaxation, reduce stress, and improve mental well-being. These activities can help improve flexibility, balance, and mind-body connection, providing a holistic approach to fitness.

7. Customization and Progression: Tailor your workout program to your specific goals, fitness level, and preferences. Gradually increase the intensity, duration, or weights used to continually challenge your body and promote progress. Periodically reassess and adjust your program to avoid plateaus and keep your workouts engaging and effective.

8. Recovery and Rest: Allow adequate time for recovery and rest between workouts. This includes getting enough sleep, incorporating active recovery days, and listening to your body's cues. Recovery is essential for muscle repair and growth, preventing overtraining, and minimising the risk of injury.

9. Nutrition and Hydration: Remember that exercise and nutrition go hand in hand. Fuel your body with a well-balanced diet that includes lean proteins, complex carbohydrates, healthy fats, and an abundance of fruits and vegetables. Stay hydrated before, during, and after workouts to support optimal performance and recovery.

10. Consistency and Progress Tracking: Consistency is key for achieving desired results. Stay committed to your workout program and make it a regular part of your lifestyle. Keep track of your workouts, progress, and achievements to stay motivated and monitor your improvements.

Supplements for Women

Supplements can play a supportive role in women's fitness journeys, providing additional nutrients and aiding in achieving specific health and fitness goals. While a well-rounded diet should always be the foundation, certain supplements can help address nutritional gaps or enhance performance. Here are some key supplements commonly used by women:

1. Multivitamins: A high-quality multivitamin can help fill nutrient deficiencies and support overall health. Look for a formulation specifically designed for women that includes essential vitamins and minerals like vitamin D, calcium, iron, and B vitamins.

2. Omega-3 Fatty Acids: Omega-3 fatty acids, such as those found in fish oil supplements, provide numerous benefits for women. They support heart health, brain function, joint health, and may help alleviate symptoms of menstrual discomfort.

3. Protein Powders: Protein powders can be beneficial for women looking to increase their protein intake, support muscle recovery and growth, or manage weight. Choose from various sources like whey protein, plant-based protein (pea, hemp, rice), or collagen protein based on dietary preferences and goals.

4. Calcium and Vitamin D: Calcium is crucial for maintaining bone health, and vitamin D aids in its absorption. Many women require additional calcium and vitamin D supplementation, especially during pregnancy, menopause, or if dietary intake is insufficient.

5. Iron: Iron is essential for transporting oxygen in the blood and preventing iron-deficiency anemia. Women, particularly those with heavy menstrual periods, may need iron supplementation to meet their needs. Consult with a healthcare professional to determine if iron supplementation is necessary.

6. B Vitamins: B vitamins play vital roles in energy production, metabolism, and hormone regulation. Vitamin B12 is particularly important for vegetarians and vegans who may have limited dietary sources. B-complex supplements provide a combination of B vitamins.

7. Pre-Workout Supplements: Pre-workout supplements can boost energy levels, focus, and endurance during workouts. They often contain ingredients like caffeine, beta-alanine, creatine, or branched-chain amino acids (BCAAs). Carefully read labels and consider personal tolerance and fitness goals before incorporating pre-workout supplements.

8. Probiotics: Probiotic supplements support gut health and digestion by promoting the growth of beneficial gut bacteria. They may help alleviate digestive issues and support a healthy immune system. Look for a variety of bacterial strains and consult with a healthcare professional for specific recommendations.

9. Collagen: Collagen supplements have gained popularity for their potential benefits to skin, hair, nails, and joint health. Collagen is a protein that supports connective tissues and can help maintain healthy skin elasticity and joint function.

10. Adaptogens and Herbal Supplements: Adaptogens like ashwagandha, rhodiola, or maca root are believed to help the body adapt to stress and promote overall well-being. Herbal supplements such as green tea extract, turmeric, or milk thistle may offer antioxidant, anti-inflammatory, or liver-supporting properties.

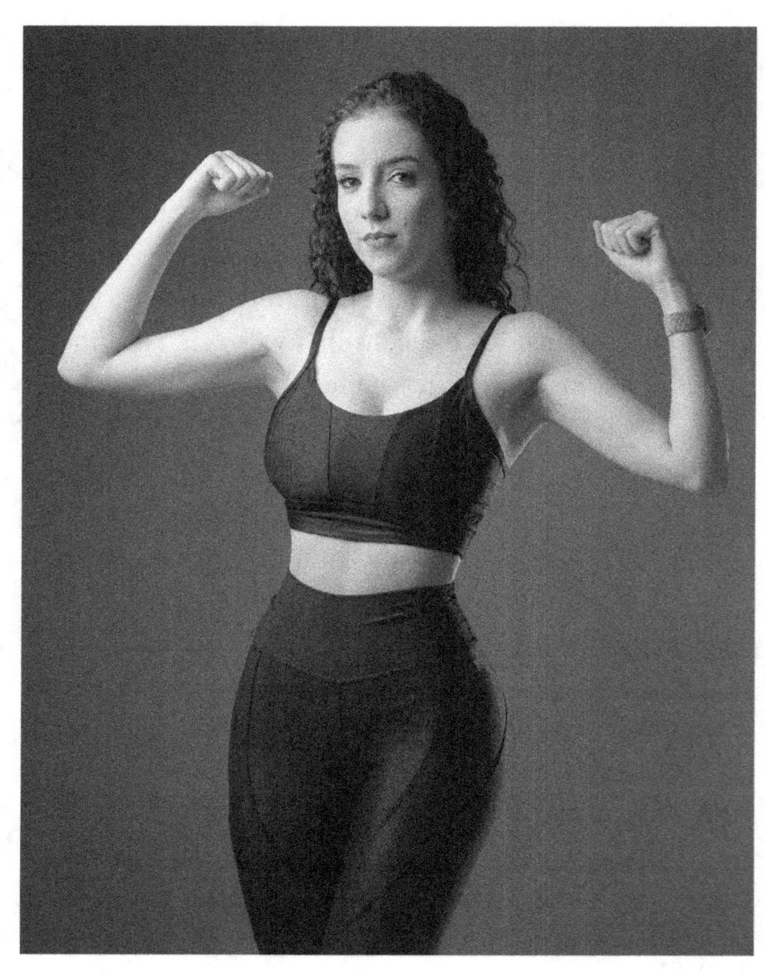

Overcoming Challenges

Embarking on a fitness journey, including bodybuilding and adopting a healthy lifestyle, can present various challenges along the way. However, with the right mindset and strategies, you can overcome these obstacles and stay on track towards reaching your goals. Here are some common challenges and tips to help you overcome them:

1. Lack of Motivation: It's normal to experience fluctuations in motivation, but it's crucial to find ways to stay inspired. Set clear and realistic goals, remind yourself of the reasons why you started, and visualise the benefits you will gain from achieving them. Surround yourself with supportive and like-minded individuals who can help keep you motivated.

2. Time Constraints: Busy schedules and competing priorities can make it challenging to find time for workouts and meal preparation. Plan your week in advance, schedule your workouts like important appointments, and make them a non-negotiable part of your routine. Look for time-saving strategies, such as meal prepping or finding shorter, high-intensity workouts that fit your schedule.

3. Plateaus: Progress may slow down or stall at certain points in your journey, known as plateaus. To overcome plateaus, consider changing your workout routine, increasing the intensity or volume of your exercises, incorporating new exercises or training techniques, or seeking guidance from a fitness professional. Remember that plateaus are a normal part of the process, and persistence is key.

4. Self-Doubt and Negative Self-Talk: Negative self-talk can hinder progress and undermine confidence. Practice positive affirmations, focus on your strengths and achievements, and surround yourself with positive influences. Challenge negative thoughts with evidence of your progress and remind yourself that you are capable of overcoming obstacles.

5. Lack of Support: Some people may not understand or support your fitness goals. Seek out a support network of friends, family, or like-minded individuals who share similar aspirations. Join fitness communities or online forums where you can find encouragement, advice, and accountability. Remember, your journey is unique, and it's important to prioritise your own well-being.

6. Injury or Physical Limitations: Injuries or physical limitations can be setbacks, but they don't have to derail your progress completely. Consult with a healthcare professional or physical therapist to develop a modified exercise plan that accommodates your needs. Focus on rehabilitation and incorporate exercises that promote mobility and strengthen unaffected areas.

7. Mental and Emotional Challenges: Fitness journeys can sometimes trigger mental and emotional challenges. Practice self-care, prioritise rest and recovery, and incorporate stress-management techniques like meditation or journaling. Seek professional help if needed to address any underlying mental health concerns.

8. Nutrition and Food Temptations: Sticking to a nutritious diet can be challenging when faced with tempting food choices. Plan your meals and snacks in advance, create a supportive food environment by keeping unhealthy options out of sight, and find healthier alternatives to satisfy cravings. Allow yourself occasional indulgences in moderation to maintain balance.

9. Lack of Progress Tracking: Without tracking your progress, it can be difficult to see how far you've come. Keep a journal or use apps to record your workouts, measurements, and achievements. Celebrate milestones along the way, whether it's reaching a new personal best or fitting into a smaller clothing size. Progress tracking can serve as a powerful motivator.

10. Perfectionism and All-or-Nothing Mentality: Striving for perfection can lead to feelings of failure and frustration. Embrace a flexible and realistic approach to your fitness journey. Remember that consistency, even with occasional setbacks, is more important than perfection. Celebrate small victories and focus on long-term progress rather than instant results.

Staying Consistent and Building a Lifestyle

Consistency is key when it comes to achieving long-term success in bodybuilding and maintaining a healthy lifestyle. Building healthy habits and transforming your fitness journey into a sustainable lifestyle requires dedication, perseverance, and a mindful approach. Here are some strategies to help you stay consistent and build a lifestyle that supports your goals:

1. Set Realistic and Sustainable Goals: Start by setting realistic and achievable goals that align with your aspirations and current lifestyle. Break them down into smaller milestones to track your progress along the way. Avoid setting overly ambitious goals that may lead to frustration or burnout. Remember, building a healthy lifestyle is a marathon, not a sprint.

2. Create a Routine: Establish a regular routine that incorporates your workouts, meal planning, and self-care activities. Designate specific times for exercise, meal preparation, and rest. Consistency thrives in a structured environment, and having a routine makes it easier to prioritise your health and fitness goals amidst other responsibilities.

3. Find Activities You Enjoy: Engaging in activities you genuinely enjoy can help you stay consistent and make your fitness journey more enjoyable. Explore different forms of exercise, such as weightlifting, group fitness classes, outdoor activities, or sports, to discover what resonates with you. When you look forward to your workouts, it becomes easier to stay committed.

4. Make Fitness a Priority: Treat your fitness journey as a priority rather than an afterthought. Schedule your workouts in advance and treat them as non-negotiable appointments. Avoid cancelling or rescheduling them unless absolutely necessary. By prioritising your health and fitness, you send a powerful message to yourself and others that your well-being matters.

5. Accountability and Support: Seek accountability and support from friends, family, or like-minded individuals. Share your goals with trusted individuals who can hold you accountable and provide encouragement. Consider joining fitness communities, online forums, or workout groups where you can connect with individuals who share similar aspirations.

6. Track Your Progress: Keep track of your progress to see how far you've come and stay motivated. Document your workouts, take measurements, and track your strength and endurance improvements. Take progress photos or keep a journal to reflect on your journey. Celebrate small victories and use them as fuel to keep pushing forward.

7. Adapt to Changes: Life is full of changes, and it's essential to adapt your fitness routine accordingly. If your schedule shifts, find alternative workout times or adjust your training plan. Be flexible in your approach and embrace modifications to your routine when necessary. Remember, consistency is about finding ways to keep moving forward despite obstacles.

8. Practice Self-Care: Self-care is vital for maintaining consistency and preventing burnout. Prioritise rest, recovery, and relaxation. Get enough sleep, listen to your body's cues for rest days, and incorporate activities that help you de-stress, such as meditation, yoga, or hobbies you enjoy. Taking care of your mental and emotional well-being is equally important.

9. Educate Yourself: Stay informed and continuously educate yourself about exercise, nutrition, and overall well-being. Seek reliable sources of information, read books, follow reputable fitness experts, and consult with professionals if needed. Empowering yourself with knowledge will help you make informed decisions and stay motivated on your journey.

10. Embrace a Balanced Approach: Building a lifestyle around fitness involves finding a balance that works for you. Avoid extremes or overly restrictive behaviours that can lead to burnout or an unhealthy relationship with food and exercise. Embrace moderation, enjoy a variety of foods, and allow yourself flexibility within your plan. Remember that a sustainable lifestyle is about long-term health and well-being.

Conclusion

Congratulations on completing this journey through the "Bodybuilding Workout Diet Plan for Women" book! Throughout this guide, we've explored the various aspects of bodybuilding, nutrition, goal-setting, workouts, supplements, and overcoming challenges. By delving into these topics, you've gained valuable insights and tools to support your bodybuilding endeavours and cultivate a healthy lifestyle.

Remember, bodybuilding is not just about physical transformation; it's a holistic approach that encompasses mental strength, discipline, and self-care. It's about embracing the journey and making sustainable changes that benefit your overall well-being.

As you move forward, keep in mind that progress is not always linear. You may encounter setbacks, plateaus, or moments of self-doubt, but it's essential to stay committed and resilient. Embrace challenges as opportunities for growth, and remember that small, consistent steps lead to significant transformations over time.

Building a healthy lifestyle is a lifelong endeavor. It requires continuous learning, adapting to change, and finding a balance that works for you. Listen to your body, prioritise self-care, and remember that your well-being is the foundation of your success.

Stay connected with your support system, whether it's friends, family, or like-minded individuals who share your goals. Seek inspiration from their stories, offer support in return, and celebrate each other's achievements.

Finally, always remember that you are capable of achieving whatever you set your mind to. Believe in yourself, trust the process, and never underestimate the power of consistency and dedication.

Now, it's time to take what you've learned and put it into action. Embrace the challenges, celebrate the victories, and enjoy the incredible transformation that awaits you on your bodybuilding and fitness journey.

Wishing you strength, resilience, and a lifetime of health and happiness.

Best of luck on your bodybuilding adventure!